Weight Loss Cookbook

Mediterranean Diet for Lasting Weight Loss

LELA GIBSON

CONTENTS

Introduction

I want to thank you and congratulate you for buying the book, *"Weight Loss Cookbook: Mediterranean Diet for Lasting Weight Loss."*

This book has actionable information on how to use the Mediterranean diet for sustainable weight loss.

Currently, it is difficult to ignore the numerous diseases and the increase in health risks that have come up due to our modern way of life. One of the things that health experts and nutritionists agree on is that there is an indisputable link between food and health. This essentially means that if we are to live a healthy life, we must be deliberate by eating healthy.

From the above explanation, it clearly means something is wrong with our diet. As such, if we are to reverse our health problems, we MUST be deliberate by eating like some of the healthiest people in the world. This has nothing to do with dieting in the sense of crash dieting but is a complete lifestyle change, which is guaranteed to transform your life for good.

The Mediterranean diet is one of the healthiest diets the world over owing to the fact that the Mediterranean people are some of the healthiest people. To help you to follow the diet like the Mediterranean people with ease, this book will walk you through the diet by discussing everything you need to know about the diet and how to use it to attain maximum weight loss and optimal health. Let's begin.

Thanks again for buying this book. I hope you enjoy it!

Before we get to a point of understanding how to follow the Mediterranean diet to lose weight and derive various other benefits, let's start by understanding what the Mediterranean diet is all about.

Mediterranean Diet: A Comprehensive Background

What Is It?

In its simplest terms, the Mediterranean diet is basically a heart-healthy diet that is based on the cooking styles and the traditional foods embraced by countries that border the Mediterranean Sea such as Spain, Italy and Greece.

The keyword is 'traditional.' This is because there have been many changes to the Mediterranean diet over the years. Nowadays, it is not unusual to picture lasagna, jumbo sized pizzas, long loaves of bread and sandwiches, racks of lamb and overflowing glasses of wine whenever someone mentions the Mediterranean diet. In fact, Mediterranean countries such as France and Italy are often associated with wine and pizza. The kind of Mediterranean diet that we are referring to emphasizes on the intake of local, traditional foods depending on their seasonality of such foods like olive oil, spices, legumes, whole grains, vegetables and fruit. You are also allowed to take a moderate amount of red wine, poultry, sugar and salt.

What you need to understand is that when it comes to the Mediterranean diet, what you eat is just as important as how many times you eat it. All that is anchored in the various components of the Mediterranean diet some of which we will discuss next.

1: Foundation

The Mediterranean diet is built on a foundation of family, friendship and physical activity. It is not just about eating certain foods and being done with it. It is also about taking your time to enjoy both the food and the company. The diet emphasizes things such as rest and relaxation. Thus, you will not only be eating good food but you will also find time to relax and unwind. These are definitely recipes for good health.

Another thing the diet emphasizes is physical activity. The Mediterranean lifestyle often involves a lot of walking and cycling. Thus, if you intend to do the diet, you need to incorporate physical activity. You can't just choose to engage in one part of the diet and neglect the rest. If you do that, you will essentially be breaking the rules of the diet and lessening its effectiveness.

2: Everyday meals

There are foods that feature prominently in the traditional Mediterranean diet. Therefore, you need to make an effort to eat them daily. These include:

- Vegetables

Vegetables need to feature prominently in your daily diet. According to the Mediterranean diet, you need to consume 2 or more servings whenever you sit down for both lunch and dinner. Vegetables are rich in antioxidants and other protective compounds and thus you should not neglect eating them. As a rule of thumb, make sure you eat from a variety of colors instead of limiting your options. You can eat your fair share of vegetables in things such as salads, smoothies and even sandwiches.

- Fruit

Mediterranean countries often enjoy eating fruit for dessert. This is a rich tradition, as it allows your body to reap numerous health benefits. Fruit is rich in both nutrients and antioxidants, which enable your body to fight off disease. In addition, fruit is quite tasty. For this diet, you should eat 1-2 servings of fruit whenever you sit down for a meal. Another good thing about fruit is that it is often quite juicy and can help you to reach your daily water requirement.

- Cereals and whole grains

Unlike some diets, the Mediterranean diet does not discourage the consumption of cereals. In fact, it encourages you to eat 1-2 servings of cereals per meal. You can eat foods such as rice, bread, couscous and pasta.

As a rule of thumb, when buying cereals, it would be best to purchase whole grains. This is because things such as fiber, magnesium and phosphorus are often lost during processing. Therefore, eating whole grains ensures that you still enjoy the foods you love without losing important nutrients.

- Dairy products

Another thing you should consume daily is dairy. This is because dairy products are good for your bone health. They also happen to be a great source of saturated fat. You can consume products such as cheese and low fat yogurt.

- Herbs and spices

Herbs and spices add a rich aroma and a variety of flavors to your dishes. Mediterranean countries are generous with herbs and spices when it comes to cooking, as many cooks use herbs and spices instead of table salt to season food.

Therefore, you need to keep herbs, spices, onions and garlic near whenever you cook and use them to give your food that added kick.

- Olive oil

Olive oil is really important as far as the Mediterranean diet is concerned. In fact, it takes center stage in the diet and thus it should be the main source of dietary lipids. You can use it for cooking and can drizzle it over your salads. You should drizzle one tablespoon of oil per individual when you add it to your salads.

3: Weekly meals

Mediterranean dishes contain plant-based proteins instead of animal proteins. However, the diet does allow you to consume 1-2 servings of fish and 2-4 servings of eggs weekly. Fish is particularly good for your mental health and it contains healthy fats.

Another food that you should take weekly is potatoes; keep the servings to less than 3 per week. As a rule of thumb, be sure to get fresh potatoes and avoid those with weird coloring or blemishes.

4: Monthly meals

Meat is one of those foods that don't appear prominently in the Mediterranean diet. You should only consume it once or twice a month i.e. less than 2 servings of red meat. Processed meats should be consumed less frequently than lean cuts. If you are going with processed meats, eat only less than 1 serving.

Other foods that should rarely feature in your diet are sugar, pastries, candies, soft drinks and sweetened fruit juices. If you must consume them, you should do so only once a month and ensure you only eat small portions.

5: Optional

Many people get a twinkle in their eyes when they learn that the Mediterranean diet includes the drinking of red wine. Well, this is an option, not a rule. If you don't like drinking wine, you don't have to indulge in it. If you like it, by all means include it in your diet. However, you have to monitor your wine drinking. You can drink 1-2 glasses of wine occasionally. There's no need to drink wine every single day even if you can afford it. In general, men can consume 2 glasses and women 1 glass.

Also, if you're an alcoholic or you have problems with other liquor, you should avoid drinking wine. Drinking wine, however innocent, can lead to heavier drinking if you already struggle in that area. It would also be good to avoid drinking wine if you have impressionable kids or if you're in the company of someone who is prone to alcoholism.

In summary, the Mediterranean diet can be said to have 3 major parts or components i.e. the food you eat, the social camaraderie and the physical activities you engage in. If you want to fully embrace the diet, you have to try as much as possible to incorporate all three components into your lifestyle. This way, you will reap all the numerous health benefits that come with the diet. Let's discuss some of the benefits in the next chapter.

Benefits of the Mediterranean Diet

What is so great about the Mediterranean diet? Why should you switch to it? Well, the Mediterranean diet comes with various benefits. These include:

Weight loss

Weight is an issue many people have to grapple with. Unfortunately, many of the weight loss diets out there offer temporary results, as many dieters gain all the weight they lost shortly after they get off the diet. The Mediterranean diet is different, as it entails complete lifestyle changes, which ultimately bring about weight loss.

So how does this work?

Well, for starters, the diet emphasizes a set of principles/guidelines, which work together to bring about weight loss. For instance, with the Mediterranean diet, you eat more healthy fats like olive oil, take more vegetables, fruits and healthy proteins fish and poultry as well as various spices. The veggies are rich in fiber, which helps keep you full for longer, while the proteins and fats take longer to be digested while at the same time creating a feeling of fullness. Spices on the other hand help increase the body's metabolism, which greatly facilitates weight loss. That's not all; the diet is effective for weight loss, as it also encourages the creation of a calorie deficit. As well as that, while following the Mediterranean diet, you are required to engage in physical activity.

Many people turn to the Mediterranean diet in order to achieve lasting results when it comes to weight loss. No doubt you're interested in the diet. That is good but you need to understand that the Mediterranean diet is not a quick fix. Rather, it is a series of lifestyle changes you need to effect in order to not only lose weight but to also keep it off.

To fully embrace the Mediterranean diet, you should:

Embrace lifestyle changes

This is important; you cannot go on the Mediterranean diet without making some changes. Some of those changes may be harder to make than others but they still need to be made. Remember, the diet focuses on lasting benefits not temporary solutions. This means you have to work for it. Fortunately, the diet can be done by most people, as it doesn't have a lot of restrictions when it comes to the foods you're allowed to eat. In order to make lifestyle changes, you should:

-Set a goal

Yes, you need to set goals. After all, how will you know you're on the right path if you have no idea of where you're supposed to go? The goals you set need to be both realistic and measurable. Thus, it would be better to break out your main goal into smaller goals you can achieve over a certain period. For example, you can make it a goal to purchase whole grains instead of processed foods the next time you go shopping. This may seem like a small change but it builds up towards the larger goal of fully switching to the Mediterranean diet.

-Affirm your resolution

Once you decide to start the Mediterranean diet, you need to let go of all the other diets. In fact, throw out your magazines and tear up the notes you made in regards to other diets. The Mediterranean diet is more than just the food you eat. It is also about the life you live and this means you should be fully committed to it. There's no backup plan. This is it and it will succeed because it has done so for generations.

-Make time for yourself

Time is a valuable commodity. Unfortunately, many people spend lots of time on others and neglect leaving some time for themselves. This should not be the case. You need to create time to be by yourself. This way, you'll be able to focus on yourself and determine your wants and needs. Once you prioritize your time, your health and well-being will take the center stage and this will affect the choices you make. For example, instead of wolfing down fast food, you'll take the time to sit down for a healthy meal because you recognize the need to give your body the nutrients it needs.

It would be good to keep in mind that the success of any diet borders on you following the diet closely.

The Mediterranean diet has its rules and those need to be followed.

**Eat smart*

As you know, you need to eat 2 or more servings of vegetables and 1-2 servings of fruit. This is where eating smart comes in. The Mediterranean diet does not micromanage your food choices. In theory, you can eat whatever vegetables and fruit you want as long as you meet the required portions. For example, you can decide to eat 2 bananas per meal. This means you will consume at least 4 bananas in a day. Technically, you'll still be eating a Mediterranean diet but this will not help your weight loss efforts as bananas tend to be high in carbohydrates and calories. You may also decide to consume high carb vegetables such as potatoes. If you continue on that path, your weight loss efforts will be undermined.

On the other hand, you can go for low-calorie fruit and vegetables. For instance, you can eat strawberries and consume vegetables such as kale, cucumber, lettuce and spinach. These food choices will still fill up your stomach but they will also contribute greatly towards your weight loss efforts.

**Effectively deal with food cravings*

Cravings can mess up your diet if you go out of your way to satisfy them. Unfortunately, years of feeding on junk food, refined sugars and processed foods can make it difficult to ignore such cravings.

However, you need to remain firm. Instead of eating a cake for dessert, eat a fruit. Don't neglect to eat foods rich in fiber as such foods will keep you full. Also, you need to eat your proteins, as they will also keep you fuller for longer. When your stomach is full, you'll be less likely to have cravings. Once you get used to the Mediterranean diet, the cravings will definitely disappear.

**De-stress*

Stress eating or comfort eating are real issues. That's why stress is often given as one of the reasons people start overeating. When you're sad, it is not uncommon to seek comfort. Some people find such comfort in high-carb foods because they stimulate the pleasure centre in the brain. You too may be tempted to indulge in such foods whenever you have a bad day.

To overcome that, you need to find healthy ways of dealing with stress. Instead of reaching for comfort food and turning the TV on, you should take a basketball and go outside to shoot some hoops. This way, you will de-stress without compromising your diet and weight loss efforts.

Yes, it is true that the Mediterranean diet is designed to help you lose weight. However, this does not mean you can't improve your chances by eating smart. The truth is that at the end of the day, losing weight is about achieving caloric deficit. Simply put, it you consume more calories than you expend, you will not lose weight. Thus, make sure that you check your portions and go for low-calorie foods whenever you can.

Other Health Benefits

The Mediterranean diet comes with various health benefits. These include:

- Guards against type II diabetes

Type II diabetes is a preventable and curable disease. For that to happen, you need to adjust your lifestyle in order to reduce the risk of getting it. Some of the things you need to keep an eye on include your intake of carbohydrates and your activity level.

The Mediterranean diet enables you to do just that. First, it is rich in fiber. This keeps you full and thus prevents you from overeating. It also works to stabilize blood sugar. All these actions protect you from type II diabetes.

- Reduces the risk of Alzheimer's

Alzheimer's and dementia are diseases that wreak havoc not only on the patient but also on everyone who cares for the patient. The good news is that dietary changes can help you reduce the risk of developing such diseases.

How does it do that? Well, the Mediterranean diet in particular helps regulate blood sugar levels and cholesterol, as it is high in veggies, high in olive oil and rich in healthy fats. All these work together to help lower the amount of carb you ingest through refined and processed foods. Carbohydrates have been largely blamed for fueling Alzheimer's.

- Keeps stroke and heart disease away

Heart disease and stroke are categorized as lifestyle diseases. This is because what you eat and the way you live your life have significant impact on whether or not you're at risk of getting such diseases. When you follow the Mediterranean diet, you're encouraged to stay away processed foods and refined breads. You're also encouraged to limit your consumption of red meats and to enjoy red wine. All these actions keep heart disease and stroke away.

- *Reduces the risk of Parkinson's disease*

The Mediterranean diet can effectively reduce the risk of getting Parkinson's by half. This is because it is high in antioxidants. Antioxidants work to prevent cells from oxidative stress, which is often linked to Parkinson's and other diseases.

- *Increases longevity*

As we've seen, the Mediterranean diet is good at keeping diseases at bay. This in turn reduces the risk of death and enhances longevity. Improved health and increased physical activity goes a long way in adding on to the years you live.

Clearly, the Mediterranean diet is good for your health. When you eat lots of fruit and vegetables, as encouraged in the diet, you can be assured of seeing some improvements as you continue with the diet.

- *Improved agility*

The Mediterranean diet takes care of your health and prepares you to enjoy good health, as you grow older. It is not unusual to hear older people complain about aches and pains especially during the cold season or after they engage in some type of physical activity. Well, the chances of this happening can be lessened by up to 70 percent when one shifts to the Mediterranean diet. When you equip your body with nutrients throughout the years, you not only reduce the risk of muscle weakness but you also get rid of other symptoms of frailty. Also, the fact that the diet encourages physical activity will help you keep active and fit even as the years go by.

Yes, the Mediterranean diet comes with various benefits. This does not mean that it is easy to switch to the diet. The good news is that there are some steps you can take to start the diet. We will discuss these next.

How to Start the Mediterranean Diet

The thought of changing your lifestyle and starting a new diet can be a bit overwhelming. After all, familiarity breeds comfort and it can be difficult to let go of things you're used to. This is why it is important to make smaller changes that will allow you to ease into your new lifestyle. The good thing is that such changes can be done over a period of time. Once you make the first change, you can give yourself several days to adjust before you make another change and before you know it, you will have fully transitioned to the Mediterranean diet. To make this process easy for you to follow, let's discuss specific steps you should take to fully embrace the Mediterranean diet.

1. *Your cooking oil*

The first thing you need to do is to stop using unhealthy fats and oils and start using monounsaturated fats such olive oil. You can use olive oil to do all your cooking and baking. You can also mix it with balsamic vinegar to create a dip for breads. You can use the mixture in place of butter. You can also use oils such as walnut oil and canola oil. These oils are also rich in omega-3 fatty acids and are thus good for your heart health.

2.   Increase your consumption of vegetables

Many people don't eat the recommended amount of vegetables each day; they eat far less than the two or more servings recommended each meal. This is something that needs to change. You have to ensure you consume vegetables whenever you sit down for lunch or dinner. You can add vegetables to soups and salads and even pizza crust.

Another thing you can do is have vegetarian theme days. For example, you can decide to eat salads or vegetarian sandwiches at lunchtime and have theme nights such as 'Meatless Monday' and 'Salmon Sundays.' This is to help you increase your vegetable intake. As you grow more accustomed to eating vegetables, you can eliminate meat from your diet and instead turn to eating fish once or twice a week.

3.   Eat healthy snacks and desserts

Another change you have to make has to do with what you eat for dessert. You can't continue eating things such ice cream and cake. You have to switch to foods such as grapes, strawberries, apples or fresh figs. This way, you'll cut down on the carbs you consume and increase your intake of important nutrients.

You also need to watch what you eat when it comes to snacks. Chips and cookies are tasty but they only work to increase your weight. Instead of loading up on carbs, you can start eating things such as sunflower seeds, almonds and walnuts. Eat a handful of such snacks to better your health.

4.   Switch up your proteins

As you know, the Mediterranean diet only allows you to eat red meat once or twice a month. This means you need to get your proteins from other sources. You can consume foods such as beans and nuts each day. You can also consume fish at least twice a week. Other sources of protein include turkey and skinless chicken. The important thing is to cut down on your saturated fat intake. Instead of cooking meat, switch your proteins.

Fish such as sardines, herring, salmon, sablefish and tuna are good sources of omega-3 fatty acids and can easily take the place of meat. You can also eat shellfish such as clams, oysters and mussels. Shellfish are also great for both the heart and brain health.

5.   Start eating whole-grains

It is important that you move away from refined grains and start consuming whole-grains such as oatmeal, quinoa and barley. In addition, you should eat whole-wheat pasta and breads instead of consuming refined products.

This means you have to make a conscious choice to select whole-grains whenever you do your shopping. You may also have to cook your own pizzas to ensure you are using whole-grain flour. This can be an excellent opportunity to add more vegetables to your pizza.

6.   Moderate dairy intake

You need to moderate your dairy intake so that you consume less than 10% of your total calories per day from dairy.

This means you can eat about 200 calories of dairy per day. You can enjoy eating foods such as cheese and plain or Greek yogurt and other dairy products. Foods such as cheese can be added to sandwiches and salads.

7.   Introduce wine drinking

Wine is part of the Mediterranean diet so ensure to include it in your diet if you have no problem taking wine. This is because of its anti-inflammatory chemicals and antioxidants. Red wine is especially good for your heart health.

As always, remember that moderation is the key. Wine doesn't have to be a frequent part of your diet but you can benefit from drinking a glass or two from time to time. You can make a practice of drinking wine during weekends or during special occasions or special dinner nights.

Mediterranean Diet: The Social Aspect

We cannot talk about the Mediterranean diet without discussing the social aspect of the diet. As we've seen, the diet is not just about eating food. Mediterranean countries place great emphasis on social experience. This means you need to form social connections as you switch to the Mediterranean diet. Social connections are a good thing. When you are in the company of the right people, eating turns into a shared experience that you can use to relieve stress and form lasting bonds. In order to improve your social experience, you should:

Eat as a family

The first thing you need to do is to make it a goal to eat as a family. Nowadays, it is not unusual for family members to grab something from the fridge and head to their bedroom instead of waiting to eat as a family. This should not be encouraged. Each family member should form the habit of sitting down at a table for meals. This way, you can get to know what's going on in each other's lives. You can also share stories and provide comfort. When you eat as a family, you can also monitor what you're eating. It is important to monitor the eating habits of smaller kids and teenagers. This way, you can spot if something is wrong.

Family meals are also an opportunity to inculcate some principles and impart some knowledge about things such as food and etiquette. This is where kids learn table manners and learn why they should eat certain foods. When you eat as a family, you also get to share certain duties such as cooking, setting the table and washing up. Every individual should have these life skills before forming their own family.

Invite others for meals

Another way you can expand your social network is by inviting others to share a meal with you. It doesn't cost a lot to set an extra plate once in awhile. Remember, you're aiming for camaraderie. When you invite others for a meal, you get to learn more about them and share stories. This can be especially good for kids, as they will be exposed to various people and cultures. You can invite a friend, a neighbor or a co-worker to eat with you. Invite people of various ages and cultures to your home. The experience you will gain will be worth it.

Cook with other people

You don't have to cook alone. You can cook with others and use the opportunity to build healthy relationships. If you have kids, you can put them in charge of certain meals and make the activity fun for them. When you cook with others, don't just stop at the cooking part. You can start with the shopping part and share the cost if you wish. You can have a cookout and invite your friends and neighbors to share the experience with you. This opens up the possibility of making new friends and getting to know others better.

You don't need a lot of money in order to have a great social experience. However, you do need to take the opportunity to invite others to cook and share a meal with you. Take that step as you fully embrace the Mediterranean diet. Here are a few Mediterranean diet recipes to help you get started.

Breakfast Recipes

Scrambled Eggs with Spinach Tomato and Feta

Servings: 3-4

Ingredients

2 tablespoons olive oil

2 cups baby spinach

¼ cup cubed feta cheese

1 medium chopped tomato

6 eggs

Salt to taste

Pepper to taste

Directions

Place a frying pan over medium heat. Add oil. When oil heats, add tomatoes and spinach and cook until spinach wilts.

Add eggs and stir for a few seconds.

Add feta cheese and stir. Cook until the eggs are set.

Sprinkle salt and pepper and serve.

Greek Quinoa Breakfast Bowl

Servings: 3

Ingredients

6 eggs

½ teaspoon onion powder

¼ teaspoon pepper powder

¼ teaspoon salt

10 ounces baby spinach

2 cups crumbled feta

2 tablespoons plain Greek yogurt

½ teaspoon granulated garlic

½ teaspoon olive oil

1 cup halved cherry tomatoes

1 cup cooked quinoa

Directions

Add eggs, Greek yogurt, salt, pepper, garlic and onion powder into a bowl and mix well.

Place a skillet over medium heat. Add oil. When the oil is heated, add spinach and cook until it wilts.

Add cherry tomatoes and cook until soft. Pour the egg mixture and stir. Cook until the eggs are set. Stir frequently.

Add feta and quinoa and mix well. Heat thoroughly and serve in bowls.

Mediterranean Breakfast Couscous

Servings: 2

Ingredients

1 ½ cups low fat milk (1% fat)

½ cup uncooked whole wheat couscous

2 tablespoons dried currants

A large pinch salt

1 inch stick cinnamon

¼ cup dried apricots

3 teaspoons dark brown sugar, divided

2 teaspoons melted butter

Directions

Pour milk into a saucepan. Add cinnamon stick and place the saucepan over medium high heat. When bubbles appear around the edges, turn off the heat. Do not heat until very hot.

Add apricots, couscous, 2 teaspoons brown sugar and salt and mix. Cover and set aside for 15 minutes. Discard the cinnamon.

Spoon the couscous equally into 2 bowls. Drizzle 1 teaspoon butter in each bowl. Sprinkle ½ teaspoon brown sugar in each bowl and serve.

Avocado Egg Salad

Servings: 4

Ingredients

1 tablespoon of extra virgin olive oil

1 thinly chopped tomato

3 tablespoons of boiled corn

3 chopped green onions

1 tablespoon of lemon juice

1 finely chopped avocado

Salt to taste

2 hard boiled eggs

Directions

Start by mixing the chopped avocado with the juice in a large bowl then combine it with the other ingredients (excluding the tomato) in the same bowl. Mix well then serve on bread slices topped with the chopped tomatoes.

Caprese Style Portobellos

Servings: 4

Ingredients

Olive oil

Fresh basil

Fresh or shredded mozzarella

½ cup of halved cherry tomatoes

4 large Portobello mushroom caps with the gills removed

Directions

Start by preheating the oven to 400 degrees F then proceed to use a foil to line a baking set to ensure easy cleaning.

Next, use olive oil to brush the mushrooms' caps and rims, proceed to slice the cherry tomatoes into half and them in a bowl before drizzling it with olive oil. Then add in pepper, basil and salt. Allow to sit for some time to allow the flavors to soak then place cheese at the bottom of the mushroom cup, then spoon the tomato basil mixture before baking until the cheese melts and your mushroom is cooked well but make sure it does not overcook.

Zucchini With Tomato Frittata

Serves 4

Ingredients

8 eggs

1/4 teaspoon crushed red pepper

1 small zucchini, thinly sliced lengthwise

2 ounces bite-size fresh mozzarella balls

1/4 teaspoon salt

1 tablespoon olive oil

1/2 cup yellow or red cherry tomatoes, halved

1/3 cup coarsely chopped walnuts

Directions

Preheat your broiler.

Whisk the eggs together with crushed red pepper and salt.

Place the skillet over medium heat and pour in the olive oil. When it heats up, layer the slices of zucchini on the bottom of the skillet evenly. Cook for three minutes and turn once halfway through. Use the cherry tomatoes to top.

Next, pour the egg mixture over the vegetables and top with walnuts and mozzarella balls. Cook over medium heat for about 4 or 5 minutes until the sides start to set, making sure to lift with a spatula to enable the cooked portion to run underneath.

Broil four inches from the heat for 2-3 minutes more or until set. To serve, first cut into wedges.

Egg White Scramble with Cherry Tomatoes & Spinach

Serves 4-6

Ingredients

12 egg whites

10 egg whites

1 whole egg

1/2 teaspoon salt

1 tablespoon olive oil

2 cups of packed fresh baby spinach

1/4 cup finely shredded Parmesan cheese

1/2 cup milk, half-and-half, or light cream

1/4 teaspoon ground black pepper

1 clove garlic, minced

2 cups cherry tomatoes, halved

Directions

Add the egg whites, pepper, milk and salt in a medium bowl and beat with a whisk until they mix properly. Place aside.

Start by heating the oil in over medium-high heat (use a large nonstick) then add garlic and cook while stirring for 30 seconds. Add the tomatoes and spinach then cook and stir for about a minute or until the spinach wilts and the tomatoes soften. Get the mixture out of the skillet and keep warm.

Next, pour the egg white into the skillet and cook over medium heat (this time don't stir) until the mixture starts setting on the bottom and around the edges. Lift and fold the egg white (which is now partially cooked) with a large spoon or spatula so that the uncooked portion is flowing underneath. Keep cooking for 2-3 minutes or until the egg white mixture cooks through but is still moist and glossy. Remove it from the heat then serve with the spinach mixture then proceed to sprinkle with some cheese.

Blackberry-Ginger Overnight Bulgur

Serves 4

Ingredients

2/3 plain whole-milk Greek yogurt or plain low-fat yogurt

3 tablespoons of refrigerated coconut milk or dairy milk

1/4 teaspoon of ground ginger or 1 tablespoon snipped crystallized ginger

1/4 cup bulgur

2 tablespoons honey

1/4 cup blackberries

Directions

Stir together all the ingredients, except the berries, properly. Divide the mixture between two jars with a half-pint capacity.

Top with the berries then cover and chill overnight even though it could go up to three days.

Always stir the mixture before serving.

Lunch Recipes

Green Salad

Servings: 2

Ingredients

4 cups mixed greens

10 cherry tomatoes, halved

10 pitted kalamata olives

1 tablespoon balsamic vinegar

1 cup cucumber slices

2 tablespoons crumbled feta cheese

2 tablespoons roasted peanuts

1 tablespoon olive oil

Directions

Add all the ingredients into a bowl. Toss well.

Divide into 2 plates and serve.

Quinoa Chickpea Salad with Roasted Red Pepper & Hummus Dressing

Servings: 2

Ingredients

4 tablespoons hummus, original or roasted pepper flavor

2 tablespoons chopped roasted red pepper

1 cup cooked quinoa

2 tablespoons unsalted sunflower seeds

Salt to taste

Pepper to taste

2 tablespoons lemon juice

4 cups mixed salad greens

1 cup cooked chickpeas, rinsed

2 tablespoons chopped fresh parsley

Directions

Add hummus, red pepper and lemon juice into a bowl and mix well. Add a little water and mix.

Place salad greens in a serving bowl. Layer with quinoa followed by chickpeas.

Sprinkle sunflower seeds, parsley, salt and pepper. Pour the dressing on top and serve.

Mediterranean Wrap

Servings: 8

Ingredients

2/3 cup whole wheat couscous

1 cup chopped fresh mint

6 tablespoons extra virgin olive oil

Salt to taste

2 pounds chicken tenders

2 cups chopped cucumber

1 cup water

2 cups chopped fresh parsley

½ cup lemon juice

4 teaspoons minced garlic

Freshly ground pepper to taste

2 chopped tomatoes

8 spinach leaves of 10 inches long or tortillas or sundried tomato wraps

Directions

Pour water into a saucepan and place over medium heat. Bring to the boil. Add couscous and stir, turn off the heat. Cover and set aside for 5 minutes. Uncover and fluff the couscous using a fork.

Add parsley, mint, oil, garlic, lemon juice, salt and pepper into a bowl.

Place chicken tenders in a bowl. Pour 2 tablespoons of the herb mixture over it. Sprinkle salt. Toss well.

Place a nonstick skillet over medium heat. Add chicken and cook until done on both the sides. Remove and place on your cutting board. When cool enough to handle, chop into bite size pieces.

Pour the remaining herb mixture into the bowl of couscous. Add tomato and cucumber and mix well.

Place the wraps on your work area. Divide couscous mixture and place on the wraps. Place chicken over it. Tuck the sides in and roll the wraps. Chop into 2 halves and serve.

Italian Vegetable Hoagies

Servings: 8

Ingredients

½ cup thinly sliced red onion, separate into rings

2 chopped tomatoes

2 tablespoons extra virgin olive oil

4 baguettes (16-20 inches long), preferably whole grain

4 cups shredded romaine lettuce

2 cans (14 ounces each) artichoke hearts, rinsed, chopped

4 tablespoons balsamic vinegar

2 teaspoons dried oregano

4 slices provolone cheese, halved

½ cup pepperoncini (optional)

Directions

Add onions into a bowl of cold water. Set aside for a while. Drain and dry with paper towels.

Add artichoke hearts, oregano, vinegar, tomato and oil into a bowl.

Halve each of the baguettes lengthwise into 2 equal portions. Carefully scoop out a little of the bread from each half of the baguettes.

Place cheese halves on the bottom half of the baguette. Place artichoke mixture on it. Place onion rings, lettuce and pepperoncini. Cover with the top half of the baguettes. Chop into 2 halves and serve.

Grilled Chicken and Grape Skewers

Servings: 4

Ingredients

1 tablespoon of fresh lemon juice

2 tablespoons of extra virgin olive oil

1 ¾ cups of California green seedless grapes that have been picked from the stem and then rinsed

1 pound of boneless and skinless chicken breast

1 teaspoon of lemon zest and ½ teaspoon of salt

1 tablespoon of fresh, minced rosemary

1 tablespoon of fresh, minced oregano

½ teaspoon of crushed red chili flakes

2 cloves garlic, minced

Directions

Start by combining the lemon zest, rosemary, oregano, chili flakes, garlic and olive oil then whisk together the marinade.

Next, cut the chicken pieces into ¾ inch cubes before proceeding to alternate the chicken and grapes, as you thread them into 12 skewers. Then place the skewers into a large pan or baking dish and pour the marinade over the skewers until some excess oil drips off.

Next, season the skewers with salt and then grill on the barbecue until the chicken is cooked through or for about 3-5 minutes.

Once cooked through, arrange the skewers on a serving platter then drizzle them with some more olive oil as well as lemon juice.

Chickpea Salad

Servings: 8

Ingredients

For the salad

1 cup of crumbled feta

½ cup of sliced black olives

1 small red onion, finely chopped

1 chopped red bell pepper

1 English cucumber, seeded and chopped

2 cups of halved cherry tomatoes

3 cups of chickpeas, drained and rinsed

For the dressing

1/4teaspoon of pepper

½ teaspoon of salt

1 teaspoon of dried oregano

1/3 cup of fresh parsley

¼ cup of lemon juice

½ cup of olive oil

Directions

Start by combining the dressing ingredients in a medium sized bowl.

Then combine the salad ingredients in another bowl.

Next, add the dressing to the salad bowl and then stir well to combine.

Then let the salad to sit for about 10 minutes in the refrigerator to allow the flavors to soak.

Then serve while cold.

Shrimp & Beet Salad With Zucchini Ribbons

Serves 1

Ingredients

Salad

4 ounces cooked, peeled shrimp

1 cup lightly packed watercress

½ cup zucchini ribbons (see Tip)

½ cup cooked barley

Fennel fronds for garnish

2 tablespoons extra-virgin olive oil

½ teaspoon Dijon mustard

½ teaspoon minced shallot

¼ teaspoon ground pepper

⅛ teaspoon salt

2 cups lightly packed arugula

½ cup thinly sliced fennel

Vinaigrette

1 tablespoon red- or white-wine vinegar

1 cup cooked beet wedges

Directions

Arrange the beets, arugula, zucchini fennel, shrimp, barley and watercress on a large dinner plate. Whisk the oil, mustard, vinegar, pepper, salt and shallot in a little bowl and drizzle over the salad. If desired, garnish with fennel fronds.

Thinly and lengthwise shave the entire zucchini using a vegetable peeler.

Tip: Choose a sustainably raised shrimp- preferably a frozen or fresh shrimp that is certified by an independent agency like the marine stewardship council. In case you don't find a certified shrimp, try looking for wild caught shrimp – one that is more sustainably caught like ones from North America.

Now try cooling the grains- the best way to cool them down quickly is spreading them out on a foil-lined baking sheet. The surface will assist in speeding the cooling effect- the foil on the other hand prevents the seeping in of any pan residual flavors.

Dinner Recipes

Greek Pizza

Servings: 4

Ingredients

1 readymade pizza crust

20 halved grape tomatoes

4 tablespoons crumbled feta cheese

½ cup drained roasted red peppers

20 halved, pitted kalamata olives

Directions

Place roasted peppers, tomatoes and olives on the pizza crust. Sprinkle feta on top.

Bake in a preheated oven at 375 degree F for 6-8 minutes.

Chop into 4 wedges and serve.

Mediterranean Salmon

Servings: 8

Ingredients:

8 skinless salmon fillets (6 ounces each of about 1 inch thickness)

4 cups halved cherry tomatoes

4 tablespoons capers, with its liquid

2 cans (2 ¼ ounces each) sliced ripe olives, drained

½ teaspoon pepper powder

½ teaspoon salt

1 cup finely chopped zucchini

2 tablespoons olive oil

Cooking spray

Directions

Spray cooking spray in a baking dish. Sprinkle salt and pepper over the fish and place in the prepared dish.

Add rest of the ingredients into a bowl and stir. Spread over the fish.

Bake in a preheated oven at 425 degree F for 20-22 minutes.

Mediterranean Stuffed Tomatoes

Servings: 8

Ingredients:

4 large tomatoes

½ cup crumbled goat's cheese

4 tablespoons reduced fat vinaigrette or Italian salad dressing

1 cup packaged garlic croutons

½ cup sliced pitted kalamata olives

Handful parsley or basil

Directions:

Cut each tomato into 2 halves crosswise. Carefully remove the pulp and seeds. Discard the seeds and chop the pulp. Place the tomatoes with its cut side facing down on paper towels.

Add pulp and rest of the ingredients into a bowl and mix well. Fill this mixture into the cavities of the tomatoes and place on a baking sheet. Place the baking sheet 4-5 inches away from the heating element.

Broil in a preheated oven for 4-5 minutes. Serve right away.

Eggplant and Tomato Pasta Bake

Servings: 9

Ingredients

1 ½ pounds cubed eggplant

2 medium red bell peppers, chopped

12 ounces quinoa rotelle or whole wheat fusilli

½ cup chopped fresh basil

1 ½ pounds small tomatoes, halved

2 medium onions, chopped

½ cup basil pesto

½ cup finely grated parmesan

Salt to taste

Pepper to taste

Cooking spray

Directions

Place the vegetables on a large baking sheet. Spray cooking spray on it. Sprinkle salt and pepper.

Broil in a preheated oven until tomatoes are slightly charred and the other vegetables are golden brown. Stir all the vegetables except the tomatoes when the vegetables are half cooked. Remove the vegetables as and when they are cooked. The cooking time varies for different vegetables

Cook the pasta according to the instructions on the package. Drain and place in a bowl.

Add the roasted vegetables, pesto and ¼ cup basil. Toss well and transfer into a baking dish. Sprinkle cheese on top. Cover the dish with foil.

Bake in a preheated oven at 375 degree F for 15-20 minutes. Garnish with remaining basil and serve.

Skinny Bruschetta Chicken

Servings: 1

Ingredients

A handful of chopped basil

1/8 teaspoon of sea salt

1 teaspoon of balsamic vinegar

1 teaspoon of olive oil

1 clove of minced garlic

4 small chopped tomatoes

4 chicken breasts

Directions

Start by pre-heating the oven to 375 degrees F then sprinkle some pepper and salt over the top and then cover and bake the chicken for 35-40 minutes or until juices run clear.

As the chicken bakes, you can combine basil, sea salt, balsamic vinegar, olive oil, garlic and chopped tomatoes.

Then refrigerate until the chicken is ready for serving then spoon the mixture over the top of the chicken.

Slow Cooked Mediterranean Chicken

Servings: 4

Ingredients

1 cup of long-grain white rice

¼ cup of fresh flat-leaf chopped parsley

4 small chicken legs and thighs

1/3 cup of pitted green olives

½ cup of prunes

1 tablespoon of capers

6 garlic cloves, smashed

Salt and pepper to taste

3 tablespoons of red wine vinegar

1 ½ tablespoons of dried oregano

2 tablespoons of brown sugar

1/3 cup of white wine

Directions

Start by adding the whisk, pepper, ¼ teaspoon of salt, vinegar, oregano, brown sugar and wine into a 5-6 quart slow cooker. Then add in the olives, prunes, capers and then garlic and mix well.

Next, add in the chicken ensuring to nest it among the prunes and olives

Then use a lid to cover the slow cooker then cook on high for 3-4 hours or 5-6 hours on high.

Then stir in the parsley gently.

Cook rice according to the package directions 30 minutes before serving then serve the chicken along with olives, sauce and prunes over the rice.

Italian Vegetable Hoagies

Serves 4

Ingredients

¼ cup thinly sliced red onion, separated into rings

1 medium tomato, seeded and diced

1 tablespoon extra-virgin olive oil

1 baguette, preferably whole-grain

2 cups shredded romaine lettuce

1 14-ounce can artichoke hearts, rinsed and coarsely chopped

2 tablespoons balsamic vinegar

1 teaspoon dried oregano

2 (about 2 ounces) slices of provolone cheese, halved

¼ cup sliced pepperoncini, (optional)

Directions

Place the onion rings in a little bowl and cover with cold water. Set aside as you prepare the rest of the ingredients.

Mix the tomato, oil, artichoke hearts, oregano and vinegar in another bowl. Cut the baguette into four lengths and then split each one of them horizontally and pull out about half of the soft bread from all the sides. Drain the onions before patting dry.

Next, assemble the sandwiches. To do so, divide provolone among the bottom pieces and spread on the artichoke mixture; if using, top with pepperoncini lettuce and onions. Cover it using the baguette tops and serve immediately.

Grilled Artichoke, Chicken & Bacon Pizza

Serves 4

Ingredients

1 chicken breast, boneless and skinless

1 tablespoon olive oil

1/4 cup crumbled bacon

1 1/2 cups Mozzarella cheese, shredded

Salt and Pepper

2 8- inch pieces of Naan bread

1 cup of chopped artichoke hearts, grilled

Directions

Preheat your oven to 425 degrees.

Heat a tablespoon of cooking oil in a little skillet over medium heat. Season both sides of the chicken with pepper and salt.

Now put the chicken into the pan; cook for six minutes per side or until it has cooked through- now remove from the pan and slice finely.

Next, put the Naan bread on a baking sheet and bake for five minutes; when you remove from the oven, brush it liberally using Mediterranean cooking oil and top with grilled artichoke hearts, crumbled bacon and sliced chicken. Now sprinkle the cheese over the pizza evenly

Bake for about 14 minutes- or until the cheese melts.

Dessert Recipes

Apricots with Yogurt and Honey

Servings: 4

Ingredients:

7-8 pitted fresh apricots, halved lengthwise

¾ cup low fat plain Greek style yogurt

¼ teaspoon vanilla extract

4 tablespoons honey

Directions

Divide the apricots into 4 bowls. Add rest of the ingredients into a bowl and stir. Pour over the apricots and serve.

Strawberry Greek Frozen Yogurt

Servings: 4-5

Ingredients

1 ½ cups plain Greek yogurt (2% fat)

2 tablespoons fresh lemon juice

A pinch salt

4 tablespoons honey or maple syrup

1 teaspoon vanilla extract

½ cup sliced strawberries

Directions:

Set aside the strawberries and add rest of the ingredients into a bowl. Whisk well and pour into an ice cream maker. Follow the manufacturer's instructions and churn the ice cream. Add strawberries during the last couple of minutes of churning.

Pour into a freezer safe container. Cover and freeze until use.

Chocolate Almond Butter Fruit Dip

Servings: 10-12

Ingredients

2 cups plain Greek yogurt

2/3 cup chocolate hazelnut spread

2 teaspoons vanilla extract

1 cup almond butter

2 tablespoons honey

Sliced fresh fruits of your choice (like apricots, pears, apples, bananas etc.)

Directions

Add all the ingredients except fruit into a blender and blend until smooth.

Pour into small bowls and serve with fruits

And don't forget to also engage in physical activity. Let's discuss how to include physical activity in your life even as you follow the Mediterranean diet.

Mediterranean Diet: Physical Activity

Another important component of the Mediterranean diet involves physical activity. If you want to lose weight and become healthier, you must increase physical activity. You don't have to be a gym rat to do this, as there are some simple things you can do to increase physical activity. These include:

Use the stairs

Stairs are your friend and you should use them often. Yes, it is true that it is not quite possible to use the stairs when you want to go to some floors. However, this does not mean you cannot walk up the first few floors before heading to the elevator; you must make it a habit to walk at least 2 floors before using an elevator. You can also stop one or two floors before your floor and walk the rest of the way. This way, you'll get to exercise your body without paying for the gym.

Park further away

Another way you can get some more exercise is by parking further away from the door. If you make this a habit, you'll be able to stretch your legs and you'll also avoid other drivers. Of course, you don't have to drive everywhere; you can use a bus and alight before your stop to get more exercise.

Count your steps with a pedometer

If you don't know how many steps you're walking each day, it would be easy to assume that you're doing a lot of walking. However, a pedometer will tell you differently. Pedometers measure your steps. If you get one, you can have fun trying to achieve the 10000 daily steps goal. When you see how many steps you've taken, you will want to keep on walking in order to achieve your goal. Pedometers can help you to gradually increase your steps. You don't have to reach the ten thousand mark on the first day. You can set minor goals before attempting the larger goal. Remember, every step you take builds towards physical fitness.

Do household chores

Household chores need to be done and they often require you to use a wide range of muscles. When you do household chores, you have to lift, walk and stretch often within the span of seconds. This means you'll be getting a full body workout.

Therefore, make it a goal to thoroughly clean your home at least once every week. This way, you can get the exercise your body needs as well as take pride in a clean home.

You can also do some gardening, as it often involves activities such as raking leaves, pulling weeds, trimming edges and mowing the lawn. These activities burn calories and ensure different muscle groups get adequate exercise. In addition, they can be quite fulfilling.

Disconnect

In today's world, it is not unusual to see people glued to their phones when they are in the company of other people, as communication has been relegated to the digital world. Instead of meeting up and arranging to participate in some activities, people are busy chatting online. As a result, their physical health suffers.

This has to stop. For instance, you must make some changes in regards to how you spend your time. Take the time to meet up with friends to play basketball or go bowling. There's a lot you can learn about people when you're in a physical social set-up.

Also, make it a point to stop watching television for some time. You can switch the TV off for the summer and instead schedule various physical activities to engage in. This will be especially good for kids as they can expend their energy and learn more about life. You can create an obstacle course for the kids and make it a game. Hide some 'treasure' in your backyard and participate in the treasure hunt. Don't forget to join the kids as they do the activities. This way, you will all get a good workout.

Physical activity is part of the Mediterranean diet and should not be neglected. Remember, your goal is to lose weight. When you combine healthy food and increased activity, you increase your chances of not only losing weight but also keeping that weight off. Physical activity allows you to burn calories and this results in you losing weight. Thus, take every opportunity to exercise your body and keep it healthy.

Conclusion

We have come to the end of the book. Thank you for reading and congratulations for reading until the end.

The Mediterranean diet is definitely more than just a diet. It also encompasses a lifestyle that embraces socialization and regular physical activity. It is also easy to embrace since it has few restrictions. However, you do need to change your mind set when you start the diet. Take a look at your life and determine what changes you need to make. After determining where you want your life to head, take the necessary steps to make gradual changes. This way, you will not only lose weight but you will also enjoy a healthy, enriching life.

If you found the book valuable, can you recommend it to others? One way to do that is to post a review on Amazon.

Thank you and good luck!

Preview of Mediterranean Diet: Instant Pot Cookbook with Delicious Recipes

Chapter One: Mediterranean Instant Pot Breakfast Recipes

Greek Yogurt

Serves: 7

Ingredients:

- 8 cups milk, whole or fat free or 1% or 2% milk

- 3 cups water

- 3 teaspoons plain yogurt

Method:

1. Pour water into the instant pot.

2. Close the lid. Select 'Steam' button and timer for 5 minutes.

3. Quick release excess pressure. Discard water.

4. Add milk.

5. Close the lid. Select 'Yogurt' button and adjust the button until it displays 'Boil'. Whisk the milk a few times until it displays 'Boil'.

6. Uncover and let milk cool to 104 -110 F.

7. Add yogurt and whisk well. Close the lid.

8. Select 'Yogurt' button. It will be set in 8 hours.

9. Cool for a few hours in the refrigerator.

10. To make Greek yogurt: Add the yogurt into a fine wire mesh strainer. Place a bowl below the strainer. Place the bowl along with the strainer in the refrigerator for 2 hours. Serve the strained Greek yogurt.

French Crust less Meaty Quiche

Serves: 8

Ingredients:

- 12 large eggs, whisked

- Salt to taste

- 2 cups ground sausage, cooked

- 8 slices bacon, cooked, crumbled

- 1 cup ham, diced

- 4 large green onion, chopped

- 1 cup milk

- 2 cups cheese, shredded

- Pepper to taste

Method:

1. Add eggs, milk, salt and pepper into a bowl and whisk well.

2. Add meat, cheese, and green onions into a greased soufflé dish.

3. Pour egg mixture over it and stir. Cover loosely with aluminum foil.

4. Pour 1 ½ cups water into the instant pot. Place a trivet in it.

5. Place the soufflé dish on the trivet.

6. Close the lid. Select 'Manual' button and timer for 20 minutes. Let the pressure release naturally.

7. Remove the dish. Sprinkle some extra cheese on top if desired and broil for a few minutes.

8. Slice and serve.

Banana French toast

Serves: 9-10

Ingredients:

- 9 slices old French bread, cubed

- 3/4 cup milk

- 6 bananas, sliced + extra to top

- 5 eggs

- 1 ½ tablespoons sugar or sweetener to taste

- 3 tablespoons brown sugar

- ½ teaspoon salt

- 1 ½ teaspoons vanilla extract

- ½ teaspoon ground cinnamon

- 3 tablespoons butter, chilled, sliced

- 1/3 cup pecans, chopped

- 1/3 cup cream cheese, softened

- Pure maple syrup (optional)

Method:

1. Place bread in a greased, baking dish that can fit into the instant pot.

2. Spread half the bread into the dish. Place a layer of bananas over the bread. Sprinkle half the brown sugar.

3. Spread the cream cheese over the banana slices.

4. Spread the remaining bread over the cream cheese layer followed by the remaining banana slices. Sprinkle remaining brown sugar and half the pecans.

5. Place butter slices all over the dish.

6. Whisk together rest of the ingredients except pecans in a bowl and pour over the dish.

7. Place a trivet inside the inner pot. Pour 2 cups of water.

8. Lower the dish into the instant pot and place over the trivet.

9. Select 'Porridge' button and set the timer for 25 minutes.

10. When done, sprinkle remaining pecans. Drizzle maple syrup. Top with banana slices and serve.

Mediterranean Breakfast Casserole

Serves: 4

Ingredients:

- 2 large egg whites

- 4 large eggs

- 1 tablespoon low fat parmesan cheese, grated

- 1 tablespoon fresh oregano leaves

- ½ teaspoon garlic powder

- 2 cloves garlic, sliced

- 1/3 cup plain almond milk

- 6 tablespoons feta cheese, crumbled

- ½ teaspoon paprika

- ¼ teaspoon freshly ground black pepper

- 2 ounces baby spinach

- 2 canned artichoke hearts in water, chopped

- ½ cup mushrooms, sliced

- 2 green onions, sliced

- Salt to taste

Method:

1. Add eggs, whites, oregano, Parmesan, feta cheese, garlic powder milk, salt and pepper to a large bowl.

2. Layer the spinach, tomatoes, artichoke, garlic, green onion and mushrooms in the instant pot.

3. Pour the egg mixture into the pot. Fold lightly.

4. Close the lid. Select 'Slow cook' button and timer for 4 hours.

5. When let it rest for 10 minutes.

6. Slice and serve.

Check out the rest of Mediterranean Diet: Instant Pot Cookbook with Delicious Recipes on Amazon, go to: https://www.amazon.com/dp/B07578G5RB

Check Out My Other Books

Below you'll find some of my other popular books that are popular on Amazon and Kindle as well

Alternatively, you can visit my author page on Amazon to see other work done by me.

1. **Ketogenic Cookbook: Quick Low Calorie Ketogenic Crockpot Recipes with 7 Days Meal Plan**

2. **Freedom: How to Make Money Online and Become Financially Free by Creating Passive Income**

3. **Mediterranean Diet: Instant Pot Cookbook with Delicious Recipes**

4. **Alice the Superbug**

5. **Madison and Astrid's first magical journey**

6. **Intermittent Fasting: The Essential Beginners Guide for Women for Weight Loss**

7. **Chakra Healing: Chakra Healing and Karmic Awareness for Beginners**

8. **SEO 2017 for Growth: The Ultimate Guide to Learn Search Engine Optimization with Internet Marketing Tips**

9. **Psychology: How to Analyze People Using Human Psychological Techniques, Body Language Signals, Social Skills and Personality Types**

10. **Paleo Smoothies: Recipes to Energize and for Ultimate Health and Weight Loss**

11. **Belly Diet Smoothies: Delicious Smoothie Recipes to Flatten Your Belly, Improve Your Gut & Burn Fat**

12. **Keto Diet: Keto Diet Guide Cookbook for Beginners with Meal Plan and Simple, Delicious Recipes to Lose Weight and Look Good**

13. **Online Business from Scratch: The 9 Step Guide to Building a Profitable and Sustainable Online Business**

14. **Weight Loss: 20 Easy And Fast Diet Tips For Losing Weight - An Easy-To-Follow Weight Loss Guide**

33. Slow Cooker: Cookbook with Slow Cooker Recipes

34. Weight Loss Cookbook: Meal Prep Cookbook for Weight Loss and Clean Eating

35. Weight Loss Cookbook: Mediterranean Diet for Lasting Weight Loss

36. Negative Calorie Diet & Dash Diet Box Set

37. Slow Cooker & Instant Pot Box Set

38. Children Books: Madison and Astrid's first magical journey & Alice the Superbug Box Set

39. Belly Diet: The Zero Belly Diet Step-By-Step Guide Which Helps You to Lose Your Belly and Enjoy Your Flat Belly

40. Weight Loss: 20 Easy and Fast Diet Tips for Losing Weight - An Easy-To-Follow Weight Loss Guide

41. Instant Pot: Instant Pot Pressure Cooker Cookbook with Easy and Healthy Recipes

42. Vegan Cookbook: Vegan Cookbook For Beginners, For Kids And For Teens For Diabetics With Pictures

Bonus: Subscribe To The Free Weight Loss Report

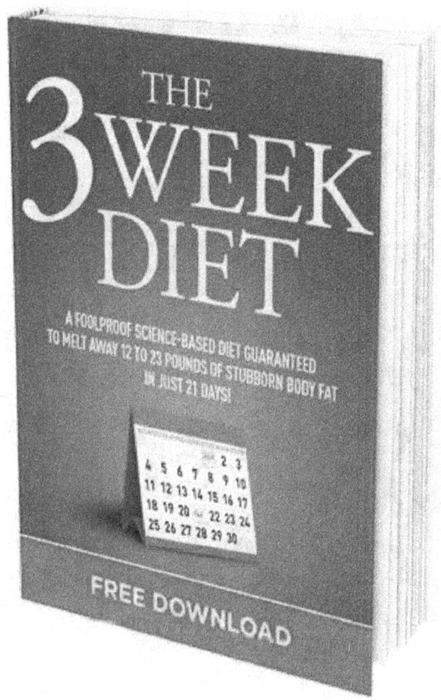

The Introduction Manual is more than just an introduction to the diet. Instead, it discusses the science behind how we gain and lose weight as well as what absolutely needs to be done to attack that stubborn body fat that, until now, has been so challenging to get rid of.

Here are the preview of what you'll get:

- Rapid Weight Loss

- How This System Works

- Why This Diet

- Why 3 Weeks?

- 21 Days To Make A Habit

- Fat Loss VS. Weight Loss

- Nutrients

- Protein, Fat, Carbohydrates

- The Food Pyramid And Obesity

- Fiber

- Metabolism

- How We Get Fat

- Triglycerides

- How To Get Thin

- Diet Overview

- Meal Frequency

- Water

- Diet Essentials

- Let's Get Started

You can access it here: **http://bit.ly/2tUb9cp**